James Chalmers

ARE YOU WHAT YOU EAT

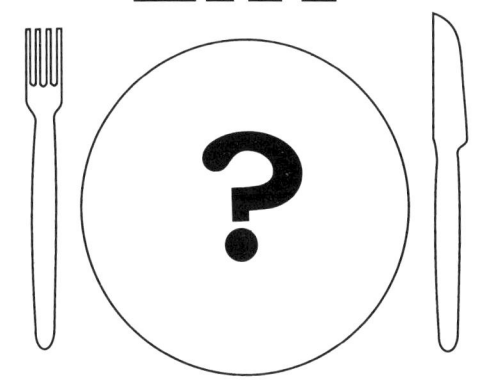

Find out if your metabolism is fast or slow - then eat the foods that suit you - to lose weight and improve your health

A Meadow View Handbook

British Library Cataloguing in Publication Data
A catalogue record for this book is available from the British Library.

© Copyright 1999 by James Chalmers.

First published in 1999 by
Meadow View Publications,
61 Greenfields Drive
Little Neston, Cheshire.
CH64 0UL
Tel: 0151 336 5979

ISBN 0 9535835 0 3

All rights reserved. No part of this work may be reproduced or stored in an information retrieval system (other than for purposes of review) without the express permission of the Publisher in writing.

Note: The material contained in this book is set out in good faith for general guidance and no liability can be accepted for loss or expense incurred as a result of relying in particular circumstances on statements made in this book. There is no suggestion that the information contained in this book will identify or treat any illness. The advice offered in this book is not suitable for women who are pregnant or who are trying to get pregnant.

Designed and produced for Meadow View Publications by
The Cheshire Art and Design Company, Little Neston.
Printed and bound by Neston Printing, Neston, Cheshire.

Contents

Preface	5
Introduction	7
Using this handbook	8
Metabolism	9
How to test your metabolism	11
Fast metabolism	13
Metabolism scorecard	16
Slow metabolism	18
Other important minerals	21
Stress and metabolism	22
Foods that cause you harm	23
Daylight and exercise	26
Food allergy	27
Changing your diet	28
Personal action plan	29
Vitamin and mineral supplements	30
Further reading	31

Preface

Just one week before I was due to go into hospital for an unpleasant test, I succeeded in identifying the cause of my problem, and when I cut this food out of my diet, within three days the problem had gone.

But that wasn't quite the end of my difficulties. I had been one of those lucky people who appeared to be able to eat what they liked without putting on weight. But now in middle age, I found my waist line was expanding and my weight increasing. Those around me said it was just something that happened when you got older. But these were the same people who had advised me that my stomach problem was also a sign of age. As I had managed to sort out that difficulty, I could see no reason why I couldn't deal with my weight problem by making other changes to my diet.

While all this was going on, I was researching for the book: *Achieving Personal Well-being.* This was to cover all the things that affect our physical and emotional health. But I found writing it a struggle, because I had lost my ability to cope with criticism. Then as my research progressed, it became clear eating the wrong thing can significantly affect how we feel, and not all foods suit everyone, because of differences in people's metabolism. To sort out what kind of metabolism I had, I devised a simple test on paper, avoiding the need for any complicated and expensive medical checks. I was then able to make further adjustments to my diet, and very quickly all my emotional and physical problems disappeared. I emerged looking and feeling better than I had done for a very long time.

I have written this book to allow me to share with you the secrets of why **you are what you eat**.

James Chalmers

Introduction

Putting on weight, feelings of depression or anxiety, struggling to fight off an infection and many illnesses, are all more often than not, the results of eating foods that don't suit us. And all of these problems can easily be put right by simply changing to a diet consisting of foods that do suit us.

Sorting out what we should and shouldn't be eating, is more involved than just sticking to the traditional healthy menus found in diet books and magazines. Reducing calorie intake hardly ever works either. People have different metabolic rates, and this means there can't be just one diet that suits everyone. For example, people with a fast metabolism can usually cope with fatty foods, like red meat, while those with a slow metabolism don't have problems with acidic foods, like citrus fruit. But the other way round – slow metabolism and red meat, fast metabolism and citrus fruit – is likely to lead to all sorts of difficulties. So it is important to know what kind of metabolism you have, before you can make the right decisions on what you should and shouldn't be eating.

Most animals stay fit and healthy because they only eat foods that match their requirements. They don't have to count calories, no matter how much food is available - they just eat the right things Included in their diets are a number of vitamins and minerals, which are essential for the metabolic process. Unfortunately much of our modern highly processed foods are lacking in the vitamins and minerals essential for effective human metabolism. Vitamin and mineral requirements are also linked to metabolic type, so this is another reason why you need to know if your metabolism is fast or slow, to ensure you have the vitamins and minerals in your diet, which match your individual needs.

Using this handbook

The metabolism test scorecard can be found in the centre pages of this handbook. Although this test is not difficult, it needs to be done with care, because an incorrect result will take you down the wrong dietary path, and this will only make matters worse. Before attempting the test, you should read the sections on *Metabolism* and *How to test your metabolism*.

After you have carried out the test, you can then refer to the section which corresponds to your metabolic type: *fast* is on page 13, *slow* is on page 18. Here you will find extensive information about what you should be eating, and vitamin and mineral requirements. Following on from this are more sections offering a wide range of important additional dietary information, which applies to everyone, irrespective of metabolic type.

As you work through this handbook, you will build up a picture of yourself and what you need to do. To help you summarise all this information, a *Personal Action Plan* is available on page 29. Having drawn up your plan, all that remains is for you to get started. Forget about counting calories, simply eat the foods that suit you, avoid the foods that don't suit you, and cut out foods that can harm you. A modest amount of exercise will help, but this doesn't have to be strenuous.

You can monitor progress by weighing yourself regularly, but your best guide is how you look and feel. Improvements can be both rapid and startling. But one point of caution - your diet will only work if you give it your total commitment. Be prepared to give up some of your favourites. Results will be disappointing if you try to pick and choose from the parts you like and don't like.

Metabolism

WHAT IS METABOLISM

Metabolism is the process which extracts the nutrients from your food, for energy and other body functions, for example, keeping bones and teeth healthy. If your diet contains the correct balance of essential nutrients, your metabolism will work at its optimum point - your weight will be right for your height and build, and you will feel fit and healthy.

If, however, your diet lacks one or more of these essential nutrients, or it includes things that shouldn't be there, this will eventually lead to weight gain and ill health. We can liken this to using paraffin to run an expensive motor car. The engine will run for a while, but it will soon end up being seriously damaged.

Our bodies are more complicated than a car engine, and we have the ability to adapt to a bad diet. It can be a long time before our metabolic engines go wrong. This is why it's difficult to accept that something you've been eating for many years, without any problems, isn't after all just an innocent little indulgence.

FAST AND SLOW METABOLISM

Fast and slow metabolism are inherited characteristics and there's nothing you can do to swap from one to the other. The commonly held belief is that people with a fast metabolism are the lucky ones, because they can eat what they like without putting on any weight. This is only partly true, because there are many obese fast metabolisers as well as plenty of thin slow metabolisers.

Having a fast or a slow metabolism depends on which side of your brain is the more dominant. (*This is the subconscious area of the brain, not the thinking part*) Fast metabolism is usually the result of left dominance. Slow metabolism is usually the result of right dominance. Some people are particularly strong either way, while others lie somewhere between the two extremes. When you use the metabolism test in this handbook, you are comparing yourself with the emotional and physical characteristics associated with left and right brain dominance.

METABOLISM AND DIET

Fast metabolisers are better than slow metabolisers at digesting fatty foods, while those with a slow metabolism are better with carbohydrates. There are also significant vitamin and mineral requirement differences between the two groups.

The physical effects of a bad diet are noticeably different too. People who have a fast metabolism tend to put weight on their torso (apple shape). People who have a slow metabolism tend to put weight on their hips and thighs (pear shape). In the UK, slow metabolism is more common than fast metabolism.

CALORIE CONTROLLED DIETS

If you reduce your calorie intake, your metabolism will compensate by slowing down. You will lose weight initially, as the body draws on its reserves of fat. But as soon as you relax your diet, all the weight you've just lost will go back on again - and possibly more - because your metabolism is still running too slow.

Calorie controlled diets don't work. The only people who benefit from them, are those running the multi-million pound slimming industry. It's not the quantity of food that causes weight gain and ill health, it's eating the wrong things, and/or being deficient in something that's vital for the efficiency of the metabolic process

How to test your metabolism

BEFORE YOU START

The metabolism test is not complicated, but it needs to be done carefully if the results are to be helpful. The difficult part of the test is marking yourself as the person you really are, and not as the person who you may have become as a result of a bad diet. For example, a person who never had dreams when they were in their thirties, but who is now in their forties and dreams a lot, should mark themselves as a non dreamer.

Note that the test will only give reliable results with adults. This means you shouldn't try to apply the dietary advice that is specific to the two metabolic types, to teenagers and younger children. You can, however, use all the other information in this handbook about foods that harm, exercise, etc, which applies to everyone, whatever their age.

USING THE SCORECARD

The scorecard is located in the centre of the handbook, on pages 16 and 17. It's important that the test is carried out honestly. Don't try to manipulate your markings to give you the outcome you think you would like. The dietary advice for fast and slow metabolism is quite different, and if you use the wrong one, it may make things much worse for you.

Start with the top line
Select either the statement on the left hand page, or the statement on the right hand page – picking the one that's the **most descriptive** of you. On this first line, your choice is between being a *jumpy and nervous* person, or someone whose *actions are calm firm and positive*.

Tick box to indicate strength of the characteristic

Having chosen a left or a right statement, tick **one** box next to that statement, to indicate how strong the characteristic is:
S = *Strong*, M = *Medium*, W = *Weak*. For example, if you consider yourself to be a **very** *jumpy and nervous person*, then you should tick the box on the left hand page, in the *S* column.

Move to the next line

After completing the first line, you now repeat the exercise for the pair of statements on the second line, and then continue down the scorecard until you reach the end. Try not to let the results of previous lines influence your judgement of subsequent lines. It is likely you will end up with ticks on the left and the right hand pages, and spread across the columns.

Add up your scores

After you have ticked **one** box for each of the pairs of statements, add up the number of ticks in each column and write these in the *Totals* boxes. Then add the three totals together on each side to give the *Overall Scores* for the left and right hand pages.

What the results mean

Overall left score greater than *overall right score* – indicates you have a **fast metabolism** – you should now turn to page 13 for the appropriate dietary advice for fast metabolism.
Overall right score greater than *overall left score* – indicates you have a **slow metabolism** – you should now turn to page 18 for the appropriate dietary advice for slow metabolism.

You can use the figures in the *totals* boxes to estimate how strong your result is. For example, if most of the ticks are in the *W* column on the right hand page, then you have a slow metabolism, but it is not particularly slow. People with the majority of their ticks in the *S* columns, on the left or right hand pages, will gain the most from the advice offered by this handbook.

If your result appears evenly balanced, and you're not certain if it indicates a fast or a slow metabolism, then you should try the test again, preferably with the help of someone who knows you well.

Fast metabolism

When the body functions controlled by the left side of the brain are stronger than those controlled by the right side, this usually results in a fast metabolism. Technically this is known as having a *sympathetic dominant* nervous system. In the UK people with a fast metabolism are in the minority – it may be as low as 20% of the population.

Fast metabolism is a characteristic you have inherited from distant ancestors, who lived in a northern climate, with little fresh fruit, a lack of daylight, and a diet dependent on meat.

It is often assumed that people with a fast metabolism can burn up almost any kind of food, and so are able to eat what they like without putting on any weight. This may be true for the early part of your life, but beyond the age of forty, the digestive process becomes a lot less able to cope with foods that don't suit a fast metabolism. People with a fast metabolism tend to put weight on their waist and torso, while their hips and thighs stay relatively slim – *apple shape.*

The main advantage of having a fast metabolism is that you are reasonably tolerant of fatty foods like red meat and dairy products. The disadvantage is having a poor digestion for green leafy vegetables, citrus fruit and wine. If you're having difficulty in losing weight, it's probably because you're trying to follow the traditional fruit and salad diets, which don't work with a fast metabolism. And not only can these foods cause you to put weight on, they can also cause stomach upsets, make you feel unwell and reduce the effectiveness of your immune system

FOODS THAT SUIT FAST METABOLISM

People with fast metabolism should have no problems with the following foods:

Red Meats – eg: beef, pork, ham, bacon, lamb.

Dairy products – eg: milk, butter, cheese, ice cream – but care needs to be exercised over the amount of fat in the diet (refer to page 24).

Non leafy green vegetables – root vegetables like carrots and potatoes will suit you. You should also have no problem with peas, onions, mushrooms.

Corn, barley and oat products – includes some breakfast cereals, porridge, and the alcoholic drinks: beer and whisky.

Poultry – meat and eggs.

Fish – all types.

FOODS THAT DON'T SUIT FAST METABOLISM

You are likely to experience health and weight problems with the following:

Leafy green vegetables – eg: sprouts, cabbage, lettuce, broccoli, cauliflower.

Fruit – especially citrus types like oranges. Also problems with jams and marmalade, rhubarb, tomatoes, grapes, wine, sherry, fruit juices, lemonade, and for some people – olive oil. But you should be OK with less acidic fruits like melon, and probably apples. As a substitute for jams and marmalade, try *Wild Blueberry Spread*, available in health food stores.

Wheat products – includes some breakfast cereals, wholemeal bread, pasta and spaghetti.

Fast metabolism

VITAMIN REQUIREMENTS

To ensure your metabolic process is working properly, there must be an adequate supply of vitamins in your diet. With a fast metabolism you are unlikely to obtain sufficient of the following vitamins from your food, and a daily supplement is recommended (amounts in brackets).

Vitamins A and E (800mcg/10mg) - recommended source is *Cod Liver Oil* capsules, but check the label before you buy, as not all varieties contain both these vitamins.

Vitamin C (600mg) - normal vitamin C is too acidic for people with fast metabolism – it can cause stomach upsets. A non acidic version is available called: **Buffered Vitamin C**.

Vitamin B$_{12}$ (1mcg) - plentiful in red meat and eggs, this vitamin is only required as a supplement if you are a vegetarian.

MINERAL REQUIREMENTS

Minerals are extracted from your food, to help build and maintain your body, for example calcium for teeth and bones. Minerals are also essential for the metabolic process. With a fast metabolism you are unlikely to obtain sufficient of the following minerals from your diet, and a daily supplement is recommended (amounts in brackets).

Calcium (500mg) - a daily supplement is advised, rather than trying to make up a potential deficiency by increasing your consumption of milk and cheese, because this can lead to an excessive fat intake.

Zinc (15mg) - an indication that you have had a zinc deficiency, will be a noticeable increase in strength of hair growth, soon after starting to take the supplement. A zinc deficiency can lead to male impotence.

	S	M	W
Jumpy and nervous	[_]	[_]	[_]
Rarely dream and/or unable to recall dreams	[_]	[_]	[_]
Like to make quick decisions	[_]	[_]	[_]
Can start early in the morning	[_]	[_]	[_]
Dislike loud or sudden noise	[_]	[_]	[_]
Tire quickly with mental and physical tasks	[_]	[_]	[_]
Intense and continual interest in sex	[_]	[_]	[_]
Often impatient and irritable	[_]	[_]	[_]
Appetite for food easily satisfied	[_]	[_]	[_]
Strong emotions	[_]	[_]	[_]
Very active and rarely still	[_]	[_]	[_]
Often feel anxious	[_]	[_]	[_]
Sensitive to bright light and glare	[_]	[_]	[_]
Can't stand the thought of having injections	[_]	[_]	[_]
Other people find your body warm to touch	[_]	[_]	[_]
Feel refreshed after eight hours sleep	[_]	[_]	[_]
Thick dry hair	[_]	[_]	[_]
Stomach easily upset by rich food	[_]	[_]	[_]
Ability to get to sleep easily disrupted	[_]	[_]	[_]
Totals	[_]	[_]	[_]
Overall Left Score	[_]		

© Copyright James Chalmers 1999

Scorecard

W　M　S

- [_] [_] [_] Actions are calm firm and positive
- [_] [_] [_] Dream frequently – often in colour
- [_] [_] [_] Take a lot of time over decisions
- [_] [_] [_] Find it difficult to get going in the morning
- [_] [_] [_] Not bothered or startled by loud or sudden noise
- [_] [_] [_] Can keep at things for a long time without tiring
- [_] [_] [_] Not preoccupied with or interested in sex
- [_] [_] [_] Seldom get angry
- [_] [_] [_] Can eat as much as is placed in front of you
- [_] [_] [_] Emotionally calm
- [_] [_] [_] Relaxed, steady and methodical
- [_] [_] [_] Often feel sad and dejected
- [_] [_] [_] Not bothered by bright light or glare
- [_] [_] [_] Not concerned about having injections
- [_] [_] [_] Other people find your body cold to touch
- [_] [_] [_] Often still tired after eight hours sleep
- [_] [_] [_] Thin, silky hair
- [_] [_] [_] Stomach never upset by eating and drinking
- [_] [_] [_] Never have any difficulty getting to sleep
- [_] [_] [_] *Totals*
- 　　[_]　　 *Overall Right Score*

Slow metabolism

When the body functions controlled by the right side of the brain are stronger than those controlled by the left side, this usually results in a slow metabolism. Technically this is known as having a *parasympathetic dominant* nervous system. In the UK people with a slow metabolism are in the majority – estimated as about 80% of the population.

Slow metabolism is a characteristic you have inherited from your distant ancestors, who lived in a southern climate, with plenty of fresh fruit and vegetables, and high levels of sunshine.

Slow metabolism means that you are not efficient at digesting fatty foods, which include red meat and dairy products. When you are young, this may have little noticeable effect. But as you get older, particularly beyond the age of forty, your body becomes less able to deal with the foods that don't suit a slow metabolism. People with a slow metabolism tend to put weight on their hips and thighs, while their torso remains relatively slim – *pear shape*.

The main advantage of having a slow metabolism is that you are ideally suited to the traditional healthy diet of green leafy vegetables, salads, fresh fruit and wholemeal bread. You should also have no difficulties with wine. The disadvantage is your poor digestion of fatty and fried foods.

Calorie counting diets rarely help those with a slow metabolism. Even small quantities of the foods that don't suit you, however low the calorie count is, will not be properly metabolised, and will stay with you as unwanted body fat.

FOODS THAT SUIT SLOW METABOLISM

People with slow metabolism should have no problems with the following foods:

Poultry – meat and eggs.

Fish – most varieties, but some people find oily fish eg sardines, and Cod Liver Oil, difficult to digest.

Fruit- all varieties including citrus and grapes, and the alcoholic drinks: wine and sherry.

Leafy green vegetables – includes sprouts, cabbage, lettuce, broccoli, cauliflower. Also no problem with root vegetables eg carrots.

Wheat products – includes breakfast cereals, wholemeal bread. spaghetti and pasta.

FOODS THAT DON'T SUIT SLOW METABOLISM

You are likely to experience health and weight problems with the following:

Red meats – eg: beef, pork, ham, bacon, lamb.

Dairy products – includes: milk, butter, cheese, ice cream and yoghurt.

Fats and oils – saturated fats and hydrogenated oils should be avoided. This includes fried foods like fish and chips, burgers, bacon and egg breakfasts. Also many manufactured foods contain hydrogenated oils, egs: margarine, cakes and chocolate. Non-hydrogenated spreads, based on soya or olive oil, are available as substitutes for butter or margarine. If you have to fry food, use olive oil.

VITAMIN REQUIREMENTS

To ensure your metabolic process is working properly, there must be an adequate supply of vitamins in your diet. With a slow metabolism the vitamins you are likely to be short of are:

Vitamins B_1 B_2 B_3 B_6 – available as a **Vitamin B complex.** A daily supplement is recommended.

Vitamin D- The recommended daily supplement is 10mcg. The best source is *Cod Liver Oil Capsules*. There are non-oil supplements available for people who have a digestion problem with oily fish. The natural way to generate Vitamin D is to have a daily exposure to sunlight on the face and hands. A winter holiday in the sun also boosts the body's store of this vitamin. Excessive sunbathing or the use of sun-beds is neither necessary nor recommended.

MINERAL REQUIREMENTS

Minerals are extracted from your food to help build and maintain your body, for example magnesium helps to repair your body cells. Minerals are also essential for the metabolic process. With a slow metabolism the minerals you are likely to be short of are:

Magnesium – a daily supplement of 300 mg is recommended to make up for any shortfall in your diet.

Potassium – not recommended in supplement form, as it is a fairly harsh chemical. Best food sources are raw salad vegetables, cabbage, cauliflower, courgettes and mushrooms, so ensure that your diet contains plenty of these.

Other important minerals

There are three additional minerals, which may be required as supplements to your diet, irrespective of your metabolic type. Many physical and emotional illnesses can be the direct result of a simple mineral deficiency. Your metabolism can also be seriously effected, leading to digestion and weight problems. The three minerals below, each have a list of foods which can provide useful amounts of the minerals. If these foods are not a *regular* part of your diet, then you should take a daily supplement to offset potential deficiencies. (amounts in brackets)

Selenium (100mcg)
Selenium is found in Brazil nuts, oysters, herrings, mushrooms. Absent in highly processed foods. Decreasing levels in the soil, because of intensive farming methods, means it is in short supply in crops like wheat, and wheat products like bread. Selenium is essential for the immune system, as well as for efficient metabolism.

Chromium (200mcg)
Chromium is found in wholemeal bread, egg yolks, oysters, chicken, potatoes, green peppers, beef, hard cheese, fruit juices. Essential for the digestion of fat, it also evens out appetite and can reduce cravings for sweet foods.

Manganese (5mg)
Manganese (not to be confused with magnesium) is found in oats, watercress, pineapple, blackberries, raspberries, grapes, wholemeal bread, nuts, tea. Helps to maintain blood sugar level and essential for proper brain function. A deficiency will often result in joint pain.

Stress and metabolism

Stress is a bio-chemical reaction which provides a rapid release of energy, by releasing hormones into the blood stream, notably adrenalin. The stress reaction has been designed to be used infrequently, to get us out of dangerous situations, and while it is switched on, other body functions are effectively shut down – including the metabolic process.

Many people find the stress reaction a stimulating experience, for example, the feeling of excitement when taking a roller coaster ride. In small doses this will cause very little harm. But the immediate after effect is a feeling of fatigue, and this can lead to people seeking further stimulation, to deliberately turn the stress reaction on again – to the point of it becoming an addiction.

Stress can be triggered by many different things. The familiar and easy to understand causes are things like a difficult relationship, pressure to meet unrealistic targets at work, driving on congested roads. Less obvious, but with precisely the same results are, for example, too much time at a computer screen, and watching violent videos.

If your diet doesn't match your individual needs, you become more vulnerable to the effects of stress. And while you are experiencing stress, it can sometimes be very difficult to motivate yourself to make the necessary dietary changes – a vicious circle that's hard to break out of. To make matters worse, some foods, notably those containing caffeine, set off the stress reaction. So when people who are stressed try to perk themselves up with tea or coffee, they are simply making the situation very much worse.

You will never be healthy and your correct weight, if you are subjected to frequent or prolonged periods of stress.

Foods that cause you harm

The average modern diet includes many foods our bodies were not designed to deal with, and most of these can be harmful. Usually the detrimental effects are not felt or noticed right away, and it may take many years before you succumb. There is also a great deal of pressure put on people to consume harmful foods, through the power of advertising. It is therefore difficult to accept that foods with a high fashion status, and which have been causing you no problems for most of your life, are capable of causing health and weight problems.

Caffeine

Caffeine is an addictive drug found in coffee, tea and cola drinks. It is a stimulant which triggers the stress reaction, and while this is turned on, the metabolic process is significantly disrupted. Prolonged caffeine consumption is also probably responsible for memory loss and absentmindedness which affects many people in later life.

In addition to the difficulties caused by caffeine, the chemicals in coffee (including decaffeinated varieties), create further problems, by draining the body of essential minerals. These chemicals can also cause serious digestive problems.

Coffee and strong tea are particularly hard to give up. If you drink a lot, you are probably addicted to the caffeine. The pain of withdrawal is worth the effort, because you will never be healthy, or the correct weight, if caffeine is included in your diet.

Naturally caffeine free herbal teas are a safe and enjoyable alternative, for example: *Redbush,* a South African tea, available in health food stores.

Sugar

Soon after consuming sugar, the body overreacts to the increased blood sugar level, reducing it sharply. This leads to a feeling of fatigue, which can be relieved by taking more sugar – this is very like an addiction. The body prefers to make its own sugar from carbohydrates, like fruit and vegetables, and any excess sugar you feed it from your diet is unlikely to be required for energy, so it gets stored as fat. Refined sugar contains none of the vitamins and minerals essential for proper metabolism.

You should avoid adding sugar to drinks and food, and always check labels to look for sugar that's been added during the preparation of processed foods. Canned drinks usually contain high levels of sugar, and cola drinks have the added danger of caffeine – definitely not a healthy drink for children. Also be aware that dried fruit and honey contain high levels of natural sugar which can be just as much of a problem as refined sugar.

Fats and Oils

The average modern diet contains around three times as much fat than the amount nature intended us to have – even higher if you frequent fast food outlets and chip shops. This is bad enough, but to make things worse, the average diet contains high levels of saturated fats (solid at room temperature), found in red meat and dairy products. Hydrogenated oils (oils turned into solids by processing), found in margarine, cakes, biscuits and chocolate, are particularly hazardous to health.

Always read labels and try to avoid processed foods containing saturated fats and hydrogenated oils. Hydrogenated oils are often present in *low fat spreads* which are marketed as *low calorie*. Unfortunately these can't help people with a slow metabolism, because people with a slow metabolism are very inefficient at turning hydrogenated oils into energy, and even small amounts in the diet can result in weight gain. As an alternative, use a non-hydrogenated soya or olive oil spread.

Foods that cause you harm

Salt
There is a plentiful supply of the mineral *sodium*, which salt contains, in a wide range of food, and there is no nutritional value in adding salt during cooking, or at the table. Too much salt places an extra burden on the kidneys. Salt is added unnecessarily to many processed foods, for example, potato crisps, which also contain saturated fat, so these should be left out of your diet.

Drugs
Medically prescribed drugs, eg sleeping tablets, can be just as damaging to your health as illegal substances. Usually, problems like the inability to get to sleep, are the direct result of a bad diet, so it makes sense to get your diet right, rather than simply treat the symptoms.

Tobacco
The consequences of smoking are always serious – premature ageing, bronchial problems, heart disease, loss of sex drive and cancer. Smokers give many reasons why they continue to smoke, but there really is only one – nicotine addiction. Nicotine addiction is extremely hard to break. But while you smoke, you will never be healthy, and neither diet, nor exercise, or a combination of both, will in any way compensate for the damage caused by smoking. It is worth while going through all the trauma of the withdrawal pains in order to break the habit.

Alcohol
In small quantities alcoholic drinks may provide some benefits to health, but excessive amounts will drain your body of the vitamins and minerals essential for the metabolic process. Too much alcohol will cancel all the gains you make as a result of changing to a better diet. If you have a fast metabolism, you are likely to find that drinking wine or sherry, even in small amounts, will cause digestive and weight problems.

Daylight and exercise

DAYLIGHT

Daylight has important links to the nervous system, which looks after our metabolism. The most obvious connection between daylight and our body functions, is the production of vitamin D - by the action of sunlight on the skin. As you get older, the vitamin D production process becomes less efficient, so this means you need to have more exposure to natural daylight

There is another link to the nervous system, via our eyes, utilising the ultra violet present in daylight. Because we can't see ultra violet, we are unaware of it's effects, but it keeps our body clock synchronised with the night and day cycle. This causes our digestive process to shut down at night, so late meals are not a good idea. Daylight, through this non-visual path, also helps the immune system to function effectively.

A daily dose of natural daylight is essential – a half hour lunch time walk is very much better than no daylight at all.

EXERCISE

Regular physical exercise improves the efficiency of your metabolism, and it helps to ensure your metabolism operates at its optimum point. The best exercise involves the steady, continuous use of the muscles, but it doesn't have to be strenuous to be effective. For example, a brisk, daily, lunch time walk is perfectly adequate. This also has the advantage of giving you a dose of essential daylight. Swimming and cycling are also highly effective forms of exercise.

Food allergy

The metabolism test in this handbook identifies foods you are likely to be intolerant of – *foods that don't suit your metabolism*. The test can't identify food you are allergic to. Food allergies can either be identified by a process of elimination, or by having a food allergy test. Your local health food store will have information about health care companies who carry out food allergy tests.

Food allergy involves the immune system, rather than the metabolic process. Food allergy is different from food intolerance, most notably in the time it takes for the reaction to happen. Food intolerance is usually not noticed until many hours after consuming the problem food (eg: a stomach upset). Allergic reactions usually happen much quicker, with the effects (egs: rash, nausea) being noticed soon after the problem food is eaten.

Unfortunately, you can be allergic to some of the *foods that suit your metabolism*. For example, a person with a *fast metabolism*, might be allergic to dairy products, and someone with a *slow metabolism*, might be allergic to wheat products. In these cases, these foods need to be eliminated from your diet, as well as the foods that *don't suit your metabolism*.

Changing your diet

A *Personal Action Plan* has been provided on the opposite page. Photocopy this page if you feel you don't want to write directly in the handbook. Start at the top, stating if your metabolism is *fast* or *slow*, then work down the page, adding notes under each of the headings. Say what changes you will make to your diet, based on what you've learned about yourself and your dietary requirements. Go through the handbook again, if necessary, to clarify any areas of uncertainty.

The personal action plan is a pledge to change to a healthy lifestyle – so start your new diet right away.

It can take up to four weeks before you'll notice any benefits from the dietary changes you have made, and during this period, you may experience the odd ache or lack of energy, as your body adjusts to the new diet. But once you have turned the corner, you'll notice your weight starting to reduce and you'll begin to look and feel really well.

As you get used to your new feeling of well-being, you'll gain a new level of confidence in yourself, and find no difficulty resisting the temptations of the unsuitable and harmful foods that used to be part of your diet.

Notes:
If you haven't done any physical exercise for some time, and you feel very unfit, you should consult you doctor, for a physical check up, before starting.

Additional information about taking vitamin and mineral supplements can be found on page 30.

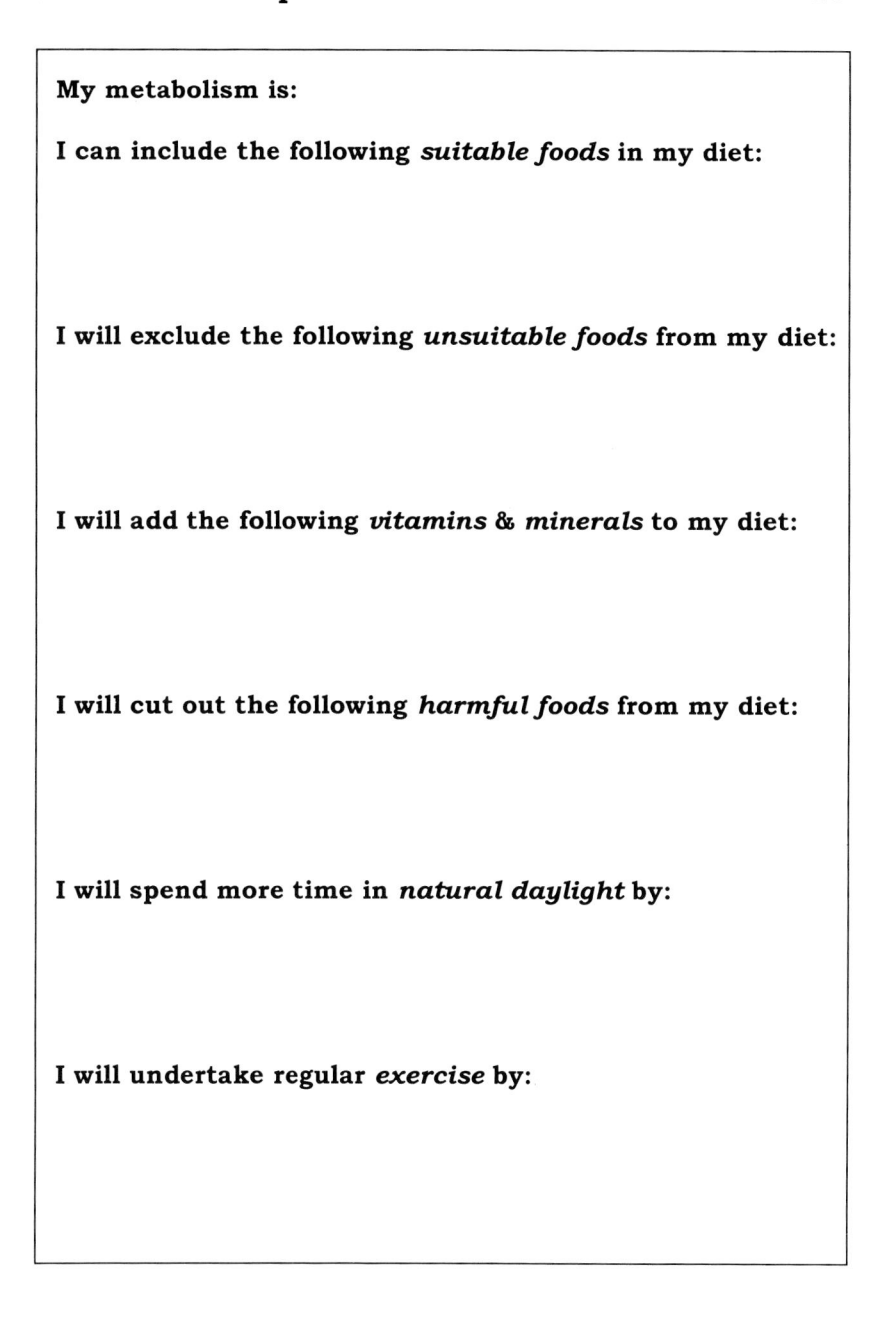

Personal action plan

My metabolism is:

I can include the following *suitable foods* in my diet:

I will exclude the following *unsuitable foods* from my diet:

I will add the following *vitamins & minerals* to my diet:

I will cut out the following *harmful foods* from my diet:

I will spend more time in *natural daylight* by:

I will undertake regular *exercise* by:

Vitamin and mineral supplements

Vitamin and mineral supplements are not like drugs. They are simply replacing the nutrients required for effective metabolism, missing from modern processed foods. The price of just a few pence per day is worth paying, because of the dramatic improvement these supplements will make to how you look and feel, when used in conjunction with changes to your diet.

Introduce the supplements gradually (eg: two per week), rather than starting them all on day one. Supplements should be taken with food. Take all your vitamin requirements in the morning with breakfast (breakfast suggestions are given below), plus calcium, if calcium is one of your mineral requirements. All other minerals should be taken with your evening meal.

You may think that taking a number of separate tablets makes you appear to be a hypochondriac, but once you begin to feel the benefits, this will no longer be a concern. Multi vitamins and minerals, which contain several items within one tablet, are not often in the right combination for your needs (except for the vitamin B complex), this means your requirements are best organised as separate and individual supplements.

Breakfast suggestions – *fast metabolism* – boiled egg (don't add salt), two slices of white toast, butter thinly spread, sugar free blueberry spread (no jam or marmalade), *Rebush* herbal tea. As an alternative to the egg, corn based cereal or porridge (with skimmed milk and without sugar).

Breakfast suggestions – *slow metabolism* – Fresh fruit (unsweetened), two slices of wholemeal bread, non-hydrogenated spread, sugar free orange fruit spread, *Redbush* herbal tea, or small glass of natural fruit juice. Occasional bowl of wheat based cereal is acceptable, with unsweetened soya milk.

Further reading

For a more detailed explanation of metabolism and diet, and further practical advice, read **Achieving Personal Well-being** by **James Chalmers**.

This book investigates all the environmental influences that affect our emotional and physical health. The chapter covering daylight is of particular importance, explaining why we need to spend more time in sunlight, and the benefits to health from natural daylight. There is also a chapter devoted to our relationship with buildings, and the places we live and work in, including the reasons why bad designs cause stress and sick building syndrome.

Achieving Personal Well-being (ISBN 1-85703-272-1) is available through most book shops, or by mail order from:
How To Books, Plymbridge House, Estover Road,
Plymouth, PL6 7PZ. Tel: 01752 202301 Fax 01752 202331